GET THAT MONKEY OFF YOUR BACK

Helpful hints guide to a happier and healthy lifestyle
Helpful guide to stress and self-esteem

by
Debra J. Fleming

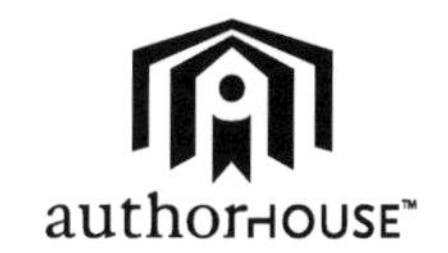

authorHOUSE™
1663 Liberty Drive, Suite 200
Bloomington, Indiana 47403
(800) 839-8640
www.AuthorHouse.com

First published by AuthorHouse 11/23/05

ISBN: 1-4208-9317-3(sc)

Printed in the United States of America
Bloomington, Indiana

This book is printed on acid-free paper.

PREFACE

This book is designed to get you motivated and make you fell good about yourself and know that your not alone and you can succeed at losing weight .in this book you will find many different helpful hints to help you along your way. I mentioned there is different vitamin you can take that will help keep you strong and put the vitamins back you work out while exercising. Always get a doctor's approval before starting any diet or exercise program. If your not healthy to begin with , you'll have to get healthy first .than you can start your program.

There are many ways to relive stress and boost your self -esteem so find the one's right for you and practice them every day. Make you mind as healthy as your body. you will be a better and happier person when you finish your diet . I practice mine in front of a mirror and it helps motivate me and helps me to deal with every day ups and downs. Always take pride in your self and what you do. Be sure and give yourself quality time, just you and no one else. That's the time you get to relax and say " aaaaahhhhh" what a day and I handled it great.

Allow your self at least 8 hours of sleep a night. You'll wake up feeling young and refreshed the next day. Remember these helpful hints throughout the book. Practice self-esteem, stress reliever exercises, don't forget regular exercising for your body. Check blood pressure and weigh only 2 times a week. You will do fine and family will be amassed you did it all on your own to start out you will be sore, but it gets easier as you go. . before you know it you'll be running a marathon. my prayers are with you and good luck. Make yourself a winner today.

Introduction

This book was designed to be a helpful guide to a new healthier and happier you. In it you will find different ways to help you get started on a healthy diet. there is helpful information on how you can get started on your diet. Included is samples of recipes, exercising tips, stress reducing steps, and a way to help with your self-esteem. All of what you will be reading is based on my own personal experiences and how I found a way to over come the fears of dieting and be a healthier and happier person. This book is dedicated to all the people who need some help and guidance, to let them know that their not alone in there search for a better way of life.

Dedicated to you, the dieters
God bless and good luck

Contents

Chapter 1
Get that monkey off your back

This book is a way to show you and help you how to eat right, exercise, and to help you have a healthy lifestyle. This is only a guide to get you started on how to get the monkey off your back and not give into it. Most dieter's don't even know that they have (a monkey) so tho speak on their back. The term monkey on your back is when you reach for that bowl of chocolate pudding, or candy bar late at night, when your suppose to be sleeping. . it's the one thing or food that you give into when something goes wrong and you feel the need to cheat on your diet.

I am speaking out of the voice of experience. My monkey is chocolate candy and peanut butter, and or any sweets in the house after bed time. When

I feel stressed, worried, or down right angry and have an upset or insecurity in my daily life. I turn to my monkey food or comfort food. Most of the time it's peanut butter and or chocolate, therefore is my down-fall or "monkey on my back". Once you give into it you feel guilty and you get an upset stomach, which in turn you get heart burn from hell. Than you can't sleep and you toss and turn till morning light.

Once you establish what you are craving, you have to learn how not to give into it. It is also known as comfort foods. Believe me comfort foods are your worse enemy and you'll never be able to lose the weight you need. I am going to help you learn how to defeat those bad cravings and how not to give into them. That so called monkey on your back. I am currently still working on my diet and it's slow going, but it's coming off slowly and will stay off. When you reach your goals you'll be very happy with your results.

You don't need a lot of fancy pills, or weight equipment, or videos. You need to find that one thing that will motivate you and stay by it until you reach your ideal weight goal. Be realistic about your short and long term goals. That way you will not get easily discouraged. if you don't het there fast enough that's alright. You can plan on losing 2-4 pounds a week. It will take time to get there so figure on a slow steady pace and soon enough you'll start seeing a new you.

Chapter 2

Stay away from comfort foods

Here is a sample list of comfort foods to stay away from when those pesky midnight cravings hit you. If you give into them you'll just be making you mid section grow and you will develop serious health problems.

1. *Cookies of any kind*
2. *Peanut butter*
3. *ice cream and toppings*
4. *Candy bars of any kind*
5. *Potato chips and dips of any kind*
6. *Pies and cakes with topping, frosting*
7. *Sugar snacks and chocolate*
8. *Fried foods cooked in fatty grease or lard*
9. *Fast foods or microwave foods*
10. *Left overs(especially fried)*

These are just a few that I have mentioned and have to guard against myself. All of these things are full of fats and sugars and when you eat them, well you are what you eat .lets talk a little about sugars and fats in the blood stream . When you eat , lets say a piece of cake. The sugar you put in it plus the sugar from the frosting goes into the blood stream . Your body turns that sugar into fat and the fat deposits go into the veins that carries your blood throughout your system. Some where traveling through the veins the fat cells get hung up and start to build up causing the vein to clog. This will cause the blood flow to slow down .when that happens it makes your heart work harder to push the blood through and causes the heart to enlarge. So if you have to have a midnight snack , try eating an apple or light plain salad .you can also drink a glass of water using a straw and then go back to bed. It will take the food cravings you thought you had away and you'll sleep better.

Never go to bed on a full stomach because it will cause indigestion and discomfort than you will be up all night being miserable. You will not be able to digest your food and than it sits there like a heavy weight. The food that sits there on your stomach will break down into sugar and than goes to a storage bend in your body. Your body stores all that extra sugar and therefore turns into fat. You need to stay active in order for you to use up that stored fat or sugar. That's where exercise comes in at. You also store it while you sleep so you can have energy for the next day. The sugar you don't burn in your daily activities sits there and you continue to get bigger and bigger. This action will cause you to gain that weight you tried so hard to work off.

Like any muscle the more you work it the bigger it gets. So lets work on not storing extra sugar so that your heart stays a normal size. heart problems can develop with over weight people and can effect over weight children as well. you can get high blood pressure that can cause serious problems as well as other physical problems in the shoulders and back. Another thing that causes high blood pressure is stress related things. For example, stressing about bills, what you'll wear next, getting kids off to school in time, worrying about every day stuff in your life you have no control over .another problem with this is developing high cholesterol. In your diet plan you need to learn what is good cholesterol and bad cholesterol.

You can control both high blood pressure and cholesterol in learning what to eat and how much to eat. Be sure and get enough exercise through out your day. There are many types of medications you can get to help you with high blood pressure and help lower high cholesterol. 'Now for a little surprise' it's alright to treat yourself to one of your favorite junk foods, but only twice a month. If you feel the need to cheat a little on your diet, do it up in the day so maybe you'll have enough time to exercise it off .Remember you want to burn calories and fat so stick to your plan and goals you have made. you can also get a diet buddy to help you when your feeling the need to cheat. Just call them up and have a nice conversation and before you know it the food craving is gone .it's a good way to keep up with family news. Also be sure and get your doc's approval before starting any diet plan. Don't want no problems or the ol, ticker giving out to soon.

Chapter 3

Midnight binging:
Dont let the midnight binge monster get you!

I have learned from past experience how to curve the midnight binges. I am going to give you a few hints on how to beat the binge monster. About one hour before bed time, fix you up a snack tray of raw vegetables and use low fat carbohydrate dips. Eat slowly , take time to chew your food. After about five minuets drink some water and you'll fill up faster and won't eat as much. When you wake up later drink some water or non-fat milk and go back to bed.

Try having a power nutrition bar and non-fat milk. You can drink water, non-fat milk , juice or decafe tea or coffee. Try to drink water slowly through a straw and surprising enough you'll get full that way too. You won't get the heart burn associated with eating at bed time or when you get up during the night. The water you drink purifies your blood stream and gets rid of the daily toxins that you consume . Therefore water is very healthy and you need to drink at least 6-8 glasses of water a day. I know this works I have tried it myself and I wake up in a much better mood. I am also ready to face the day. I feel like taking on what ever comes my way every day.you also don't get as stressed as you normally would.

You can choose from an assortment of vegetables or fruits for a midnight snack. You can eat them raw or prepare them cooked and then warm them up. Some of my favorite fruits and veggie are peaches, apples,, pears plums,. Some of my favorite veggie are lettuce, celery, broccoli, tomatoes, . Some of these foods you can have different types of your favorite dips. Ranch Italian, oil and vinegar, ... with your fruits you can have lite whipped cream, lite caramel, lite chocolate. This way you get your sweet tooth taken care of and you can stay on your diet and not feel guilty. "Even if you like grandma's favorite left overs, don't midnight binge on them"

→ ***You love grandma's cooking her weight in gold, don't binge*** ←

Chapter 4

Exercise that monkey away

Like with any diet you have to exercise some or it takes longer to lose weight. Set yourself a short and long term goal to lose the weight. Br sure and I stress again get your doctor's approval before starting any diet or exercise plan. it's always good to start with aa clean bill of health before exercising. Exercising is important to help you to lose the weight and to help tone up your muscles as you begin to lose weight. As you start to exercise you will build muscle first. " so don't get discouraged ' before you begin. Don't give up the weight will start falling off before you know it. Start off with a low impact exercise program one that fits your needs. Work your way up as each set gets easier, than move to a more advanced exercise program. make your exercising fun, invite a friend and just have fun. You won't get board as fast that way.

I have found out that walking, bike riding, even playing some sort of ball game is exercise too, it's also fun and you stay active. You also get to be out doors and not have to stay in hidden from the world. A few more fun ways to lose weight and burn those calories is to go swimming or dancing. Who wouldn't enjoy a night out for fun. Guess what most people don't think of this one, "having sex will burn 250 calories up fast, so enjoy yourself and fun with your partner. It's one of America's favorite past times.

If your one of those people that just want the equipment than buy the ones that will help you lose weight in those target areas that you want to tone up. You can use a towel in place of a thera band. This method is to exercise your arms and it doesn't hurt as much. When you place the towel behind the head, you pull one way than you pull another, you are creating resistance and work the arm muscles. This is the way to get rid of the "bye, bye, flap" as I like to call it. It's the extra skin you have when you raise your arm to wave good bye to someone. If you have let yourself go like I have you tend to get that hang sown skin under your arm. You can go to any of your local stores and purchase these items at a low cost and is a great investment.

So are you ready to exercise yet, just find the right motivation and get the right frame of mind and go to it. My motivation is my health, my husband

and that pretty blue dress I saw at Wal-mart not long ago. I have only been exercising and dieting truly for the first time since January and I have lost 16 pounds. It's slow but a start and I feel much better. So I will keep my weight lose program up and see where it takes me in one year. If I can do it you can, because I use to be the excuse queen that there ever was.

Chapter 5

Great food for great people

You are what you eat, so choose your food carefully. Eat 3-4 small meals a day. You can have a variety of salads and fruits and if you are a meat lover like I am, you can have all white meats. White meats are chicken, fish, turkey breast, and some cuts of pork. Prepared with pam or virgin olive oils seasoned just right are very healthy and good. you may prefer to eat by it's self or in a salad either way is good. A few ways I fix my meals are low in cholesterol, fat and calories. I use virgin olive oil, peanut oil, or low fat butter or pam. The things you have to watch the most in your diet is fat intake and calories. You think it is hard but it isn't. I put myself on a 1200 calories diet and eat low fat things. I exercise about 3-4 days out of a week. This is O.K. because you don't want to over work your muscles , that leads to pain and possibly visits to the doctor.

This is the diet plan I put myself on and I will share it with you, now just because it works for me ,it may not be just right for you. You are welcome to try it to see if it works. I have ½ slice toast, 1 fried egg in butter, 2 slices of turkey beacon and 1 cup of tea, sometimes non-fat milk .for a snack I w have ½ slice of apple or drink some juice. For lunch I have a salad of my choice with low fat, low carb ranch dressing with a glass of ice tea. The tea is diet tea for another snack I have ½ cup of chocolate pudding, low fat. With glass of milk. Than for dinner I have another light salad and just before bed I have raw veggie with dip or peaches with lite whipped cream. It's a sample of how you can set your diet up and never go hungry and still get some of your favorite things to eat. I also make sure I get my 6-7 glasses of water in a day.

Be sure and get your daily requirements of milk, fruits ,and vegetables .they all play a major role in your journey to lose weight. For your confidence, I have included two of my favorite recipes I hope you'll try and enjoy.

Vegetarian dishes:

I have included a few of my favorite dishes that are very high in vitamins , low in cholesterol and fat. Prepare and enjoy the unique flavor of great Diet dishes.

No meat lasagna

1 ½ dried porcini mushrooms, chopped
1 garlic glove,chopped
1 tsp lemon juice
14 oz. Canned chopped tomato sauce
3/4 quanitiy cheese
½ freshly grated Parmesan cheese
6 sheets no-precook lasagna
2 tbsp. Olive oil
½ onion, chopped
½ tsp Dijon mustard
Salt and pepper
1/4 cup butter
½ pond white mushrooms thinly sliced

Preheat oven to 400 degrees add ingredients as you would like the layer of your lasagna to be. Cook for 20 to 30 minuets let stand for 10 minuets and serve. It smells good and kids love the taste.

Phyllo pockets

4 tbsp of butter
1 tbsp corn oil
4 leeks, sliced
1 ½ onion, chopped
Scants
12 sheets of phyllo pastry
2 tsp chopped thyme
salt and pepper
2 tbsp light cream
1 garlic glove, chopped
1 ½ cups grated Swiss cheese

Pre heat oven to 350 degrees, melt half the butter with oil in a large skillet over low heat. Add leeks, onions, garlic, and thyme, season to taste. Cook stirring frequently, for 10 minuets, stir in cream and cook for an additional 2-3 minuets, remove from heat and let cool. Stir in cheese and cover with plastic for 30 minuets. Melt remaining butter and brush a little on a cookie sheet. Brush 2 sheets of phyllo with butter and place on top of the other. Put in your leek filling and roll be sure and put seem sown on coolie sheet. Repeat until all sheets are used, brush remaining butter on ,bake for 30 minuets or until golden brown . Than serve, better than the ones you buy in the store.

This is only a few recipes that are my favorite, but you can purchase a veggie book in any book store and it will show you how to prepare these wonderful dishes. Explore with the recipes and create some of your own and have fun in the kitchen and invite your children to help. That also give you family time. You can alter some of the recipes by adding your favorite cheeses, or vegetables. If you add any meat, be sure it's white meat and that it is chopped up. You want to watch how much salt you add because too much salt causes water retention and high blood pressure most foods have enough salt in them you don't need to add to much more.

All foods have there own sugars and salts when they are growing, they get it from the water and earth. Mother nature has away of providing enough salt and sugar. Back in the old days our ancestor's didn't have seasonings they let mother nature provide for them. As time advanced we made salt. Now everyone needs a certain amount of salt in their diet so only put enough salt to season. No extra.

Remember these simple rules when cooking. Bake, broil, boil, grill, never fry. Frying foods absorbs fats in the food and your really only eating grease. If you just have to have it fried, be sure and drain on a paper towel. Than you can see how much fat and grease you were about to eat. For a small test , buy a bag of cheatoes , lay them on a paper towel for about 5 minuets and you can see the fat. Also if you take a cheeto hold it away from you , light it with a lighter it instantly burns and it's the fat in it that makes it do that. I don't know about you! But I would not want that much fat going into me .remember it all turns to fat and clogs the arteries and causes health problems,.

In your dieting remember that there are food supplements you can take , they are vitamins and helps you maintain a healthy diet. A few good vitamins are one a day , centrum, flintstone,. Be sure and find out what your body needs as far as your daily requirements go. Always get in 6-7 glasses of water a day to wipe or flush out the toxins in your body. There are different beverages you can have that are low in sugar, caffeine, and calories. I like diet tea, cream sodas, citrus juices and my water. Watch what you eat and drink and you'll see the difference on how you feel. There is shopping guides you can purchase to help you buy the right kinds of foods. it's fun and easy to use it just takes a little more time. Be a label reader that will help also. you will be able to cook a 7 course meal and all of it be healthy and no one is the wiser and you make sure your loved ones are eating right .

Chapter 6

Find out what works for you

By exploring the diet world you can pretty much find out which diet works for you and incorporate it into your busy schedule. Find out if your high or low maintenance. What I mean by that is are you a stay at home person or do you work. you can always find time in your schedule to exercise. Don't be the queen or king of excuses, you'll get nowhere. Even if it's for 10 minuets out if the day you can find time. Another thing you can do is fine a nutritionist and see what foods fight fat and eat up sugar. I find that lettuce , celery, are just two that have no sugar and there good to eat. If you have to have candy eat sugar free candy. Just about everything has some sugar and fat in it. so read your labels carefully, so not to get to much. That includes your salt intake.

Here are a few foods that will help while on your diet. Cabbage, broccoli, asparagus, lettuce, tomatoes, carrots. For the cheese lovers out there. There is three cheeses that you can have and they are cheddar, mozzarella. Swiss. These cheeses are low in fat and sugar, salt. So they are better for you. now remember this is only a short guide to help you stat a diet , it's not intended for you to faithfully stick to, it's just to help you along your way to a new improved you .now I am going to share my story to you so you can see what struggles I have had to over come in my life and to find out who I am and how to diet properly.

When I was 18 and fresh out of school, I was skinny, had long hair, and not bad looking .I had decided that married life was the best thing for me. I have three children from my first marriage and one from the second , which is still thriving. After 4 years with the first husband we got divorced. That's when depression set in and so did the weight. I ate everything I could get my hands on. The weight began to add up fast. Two years later I remarried and had one more child, plus raising three of my second husbands children. With him being gone a lot on the road, the depression set in again. My self-esteem was low and I was always tired. I got even more depressed because I gained even more weight. Raising seven children was hard work and very demanding and I felt I had no time to exercise. And I turned to comfort food. that was a big mistake.

No matter how many times I tried to diet or exercise I always found an excuse not to . My life went on and six years later I went through tough times and had three surgery's that bed ridden me six months out of a year each time. Needless to say I could not exercise so what I ate made me gain weight. So here I am today not quit as big and I am taking my life back into my hands, I exercise regularly, watch what I eat and no more mid night binging. My weight is dropping off slowly but steady. Not as fast as I would like . I have learned different things about lowering my stress level and boosting my self-esteem. I can finally play with my grandchildren and not fall sown with exhaustion. I still have a ways to fo to meet my goals that I have set for myself, but I feel I will succeed before this year is out.

So what I am trying to say is take a good look at your life. If it's not what you want"change it", you're the only one who can. You will feel better , look better, and be able to so all the things you have always wanted to do. You will soon develop a great and healthy life style and feel good about yourself because you did on your own and succeeded all by yourself. there are millions of people who have the same problems losing weight that you or I have. They just need a little help getting there. Dieting is never easy and gets harder as you go but if your true to yourself you can do anything you set your mind to.

I will tell you that I use yoga, teabo, and a n exercise machine to help me. My family is very supportive. So with this in mind I feel I can go on with this diet and succeed. Being obese can cause a lot of mental and physical problems. So I stress once again seek a doctor and get the go ahead to do a diet or exercise program. you can join groups to help you, get a diet buddy, or exercise buddy. Diet groups will also help with low self-esteem and stress issues. Everyone needs some one now and again .so don't be shy and find someone to help you through your good times and troubled times. You can be anything you like as long as you like your self in the out come of dieting. by the time a year is up people you have meet everyday will say you look great, what did you do to your self, how can I look that great. And it will be your proudest day you'll never forget.

Chapter 7
Your self-esteem

Lets talk a little about self-esteem. You either have an high or low self-esteem about yourself. I have a low self-esteem right now and have to do my exercises on self-esteem every day. I have had it since a child and one of these days I'll whip it. That's what I look forward to. I never had a good opinion of myself and what I could do in my life if I just wasn't afraid to try. I have had some people in my life tell me I was not smart enough, had no common sense, didn't have a brain god gave a goose, . But you know what I do have a brain and decided to use it for the good of myself. After a while you begin to believe what they say , so you either continue on believing or you change it and do things for yourself.

I even tried being something or some one I wasn't. That effected my whole family. I died my hair, change my clothing, my attitude. I found out almost to late it's not worth it to do that to yourself. So just be who you are and don't change for them change for yourself. I thought changing that way would be good for every one but found out it didn't work. so I am putting myself back together and hoping for the best . You can too! Always do your best and that's all you can do. the one person I thought I was helping in doing this little change , I found out was hurting them . So you make the descion to try and change for the better. And some how it works out for you .I took a long hard look into myself and decide I would be the person I was born to be and let the rest fall into play. Now I am glad I did.

So always be true to yourself and don't change for anyone but yourself. You'll be happy you did. I have compiled a list of positive things for you to work on while your on the way to self discovery and finding the new you. Hopefully ir will raise your self -esteem the way it did mine.

1. Always think positive in life.
2. I am in control of my life.
3. I look and feel beautiful today.
4. I will succeed in my choices and goals.
5. I am smart and witty
6. I can refuse that piece of cake or cookie
7. I am what I eat
8. Will not let anyone dampen my spirit
9. I did well on my diet today.
10. Always compliment yourself daily.

Always compliment yourself in what ever you do and don't worry about little things. If you can think of some more positive things feel free to add them to my list. Above all never let anyone tell you that you can not succeed at what you want in life.

Chapter 8

Stress relievers

There are many things you can do to relieve every day stress in your busy day. many people have stress related health problems, some they never even thought of. Did you know you can run your stress level so high that you can actually explode your heart. That's why people say calm down to an upset or stressed out person. So many things stress people out. Like driving in traffic, taking kids to school, their jobs, family friends. They just don't take the time to relieve their stress. Stress causes you memory loss, chest pains, fatigue, tiredness, bad coloring to your skin, migraine headaches, you either lose weight or gain it.

There are many kinds of stress, for one I am a stress eater, when I get really stressed I eat. And usually it's the wrong kind of food. There are people who clean when there stressed, drive, or even sit down and give a good cry. Find out what kind of stress you have and find a way to relieve that stress. It can kill you if your not careful. I wound up in the hospital once , thought I was having an heart attack. it was luckily just stress and I took the stress relievers and now I feel better. but sometimes you need medical help , don't be afraid to seek help if you need it.

This list that I have provided you will help you in work, at home, or help you deal with family matters.

1. Take long walks and enjoy nature.
2. Take a nap in the middle of the day(if time allows)
3. Go window shopping(look for cloths 3-4 sizes to small it give you incentive.)
4. Listen to nature tape and relax(in hot bath, bed, out doors)
5. Go to your favorite gym.
6. Exercise 5-10 minuets a day
7. Go dancing(at home or a club)
8. Go for a drive
9. Play with a baby
10. Play a video game

This is just a few stress relievers I do every day and they work for me, give them a try you might find they work for you. Or you can come up with your own way to relieve stress. some times being by your self is a great way to relieve stress. just lying down in a quite room, listening to music or the ticking of a clock will work. The key thing is to relax from what ever is stressing you out. When the stress is gone you can finish out the day stress free.

Always take a few minuets out of your day for yourself, you'll be glad you did. I hope these few exercises will help you in some way. Remember to eat healthy foods, don't midnight binge, drink your 6-7 glasses of water a day. Get an exercise program going and stick to it .never give up on yourself because you are all you really have. I can't stress enough how important it is that you take care of yourself and to seek medical advice before starting any diet or exercise plan.

I hope that you have enjoyed my guide and that you can benefit from my advice about dieting and exercising. I wish you all the best with what ever choices that you make in your quest to lose weight and be a healthier , happier brand new you.

"God helps those who help themselves"

Your friend

Chapter 9
A little reminder

We all know how easy it was or is to gain weight , but how hard is it to lose ?. With the right motivation and training and family support any one can lose weight. I am a prime example on how hard it is to lose those unwanted pounds. When my grandchildren started saying look grandma your fat, I figured it was time. It's never to late to lose weight or tone up what you have already. First you have to decide is this for myself or for some one else. Hopefully you said yourself. Don't lose weight for some one else because if you do , you'll fail and be very depressed.

Like I said before I wanted to lose weight because I thought it would make the family members happy, all it did was create problems. Now I am doing it for myself and no one else. Because I want to be healthy , trim and a beautiful grandmother, " not to mention a beautiful lady for my husband". I weigh 210 right now and I have lost 12 pounds since February, I plan by next year to my old self of 135. Now that's a big goal but it's my long term goal. Short term is averaging 2-5 pounds in a month. Remember if it comes off slow it will stay off. Now you say that's not that much , well as busy as I stay that's a good figure.

I dance, walk, ride a bike, and exercise to yoga and Pilates. It's fun and a great work out. I hope in a few months to be advanced enough to do Teabo. . with a friend it's fun to do these exercises. Don't worry about if you look funny, your friend does to. When weighing your self don't weigh every day, weigh yourself every 2 weeks or so. That way you can see the weight coming off. you are less likely to get discouraged. When it comes down to your health and blood pressure you will stay with this diet and exercising faithfully. Because your all you have and you have a lot to live for. don't look at it like I am dieting , say that you are changing your eating habits and the exercising is just for fun.

Try this one on for size, while your sitting in a chair watching t.v. hold one leg out straight and count to 10. Put that leg down and switch to the other one. You are exercising and tighten your leg and hip muscles and soon you'll have toned up figure. You'll look great from behind in your pants.

another exercise you can do just sitting around, put your hands together and push against them , release and do it again at least 10 times. This will tighten those“ bye ,bye flaps” I mentioned. So you see there’s always time to exercise. So what are you waiting for get in there and go to work and improve or build a new you.

List of vegetables for your diet

Broccoli	Turnips	Mustard greens
Brussel sprouts	Cabbage	Radishes
Beets	Carrots	Celeriac
Ginger root	Burdock	Parsnips
Sweet potatoes	Rutabaga	Endive
Lettuce	Taro	Spinach
Watercress	Sorrel	Radicchio
Green beans	Peas	Soybean
Mushrooms	Zucchini	Yellow squash
Chayote	Artichokes	Asparagus
Cardoon	Bamboo shouts	Celery
Corn	Cucumbers	Eggplant
Fennel	Okra	Peppers
Alfalfa sprouts	Tomatoes	Garlic
Leeks	Onions	Scallions
Shallots	Tofu	Tempeh

These foods are low in carbohydrates, sugar, fat. They are good raw but if you prefer you can steam them and are really good. You get the true flavor of the vegetables and the right amount of vitamin's.

List of delicious fruits

Blackberries	Blueberries	Cranberries
Currents	Gooseberries	Raspberries
Strawberries	Grapefruits	Kumquats
Lemons	Lime	Oranges
Tangerines	Cantaloupes	Watermelon
Crenshaw	Honeydew	Kiwi
Avocado	Bananas	Coconut
Mangos	Papaya	Pineapple
Passion fruit	Apricots	Cherries
Nectarines	Peaches	Plums
Grapes	Apples	Pears

These fruits are very good and low in sugar, salt . Great in a salad or steamed add water chestnuts with the salad and favorite dressing and you have a tangy surprise.

Vitamins you can have

One a day	Centrum	One source
Flintstone	Natural herbs	Green tea
Vitamin A	Vitamin C	Vitamin D-3
Vitamin E	Vitamin K	Vitamin B`1,2,6,12
Calcium	Magnesium	Zinc
Selenium	Copper	Chromium
Potassium	Citrus bioflonoids	Grape seed extract
Boron	L-glutamine	Garlic

These vitamins are just a few you will find that will help you keep the vitamins you exercise and sweat out your body. They put them back in so you don't dehydrate as bad and you can keep up your strength. Check all vitamin bottles for the ones you'll need. Like I said be a label reader.

Exercise tapes

DANCING TO THE OLDIES OR ANY MUSIC YOU WOULD LIKE

PILATES GREAT FOR STRETCHING AND BENDING

TEABO FOR THAT GOOD WORK OUT ALL OVER

BUNS OF STEAL (LOOK GREAT IN THOSE JEANS)

You can buy exercise videos of all kinds , you decide on what area you need work on .there all good and great for the heart. Go slow than as you get stronger and better advance to the next level. The equipment you might keep in mind is hand weights for walking or plain exercising. You can use things from home like soup cans, towels, edge of cough to do sit-ups .you can even use a broom handle for helping you stretch your arms and shoulders. Either way you do it you will look and feel great in your new body.

Enjoy and have fun !

Helpful shopping guide

This is a helpful information guide that will help you with your shopping and help you choose the right foods to stock your pantry with healthy foods. There are many probably hundreds of different shopping books to help you choose your meals. The thing to do is make a menu for the week and than plan to go shopping. They will show you what kinds of food that you need that are low in calories, carbohydrates, protein, cholesterol sodium, fats and fiber.

All the essential ingredients needed to lose weight and have healthy muscles and bones. If you think about it a person needs to think about all of this in their quest to lose weight. Some say you only need to watch just calories and fat. I say watch calories, fat, and some carbohydrates. I only needed to be on a 1200 calories diet to help me plus my exercising. you need to find which amount of calories you need to take in and go with it.

You can get any of these books at Barnes and noble, Hastings, Wal-mart, k-mart or at any of your neighboring book stores.

Pep talk

Now that you have read this book I hope that it helps you in your quest to lose weight and hope my story will inspire you that your not alone and that I am just like you and we all need help from time to time. follow your hearts and keep a clear prospective on life and what it can become. Look forward to having a happier and healthier life. You only live once make the most of it and have fun!

Your friend

About the Author

My name is Debra Fleming, I am 44 years old. A mother of 7 kids and a grandmother of 15 grand kids. I have been married for 22 years to a loving wonderful man that is a truck driver. My hobbies are sketching, reading, out door activities and enjoying my family. I also enjoy writing short stories and traveling across the United States with my husband in his diesel truck. I decided to write "Get That Monkey Off Your Back" to help other people like myself, to cope with all the different stressful things associated with dieting based on my own experiences and to let them know they're not alone. If not for the constant encouragement and guidance from my husband I would not have written this book. So I would like to dedicate my first book to him, I love you Ed.

Made in the USA
Columbia, SC
17 February 2021